Unlocking the Power Within with Kegel: Unleashing Your Health Potential through Kegel Exercises

Chapter one

Introduction

There exists a hidden power in each of us, one that lies beneath the surface, waiting to be discovered and unlocked. This hidden gem is capable of transforming our lives, our health, and our overall well-being. However, far too often, it remains untapped, clouded by a lack of knowledge and awareness. The secret to unlocking your full potential lies in an unexpected source—Kegel exercises.

"Unlocking the Power Within with Kegel: Unleashing Your Health Potential through Kegel Exercises" will serve as a comprehensive guide to understanding, mastering, and benefiting from the wonders of Kegel exercises. Kegel is not merely a physical activity—it is a holistic approach to improving our overall health and well-being from the inside out.

1.1 Exploring Health: What's a Kegel?

Exploring Health: What's a Kegel?

The concept of Kegel exercises might be new to many, but it is, in fact, a time-tested practice that offers an array of health benefits for both men and women. Before diving into the details, let's begin by understanding the origin and foundation of these exercises, including the pelvic floor and its vital role in our daily lives.

Origin of Kegel Exercises: Dr. Arnold Kegel

Kegel exercises owe their name to Dr. Arnold Kegel, an American gynaecologist who first proposed these exercises in the 1940s as a non-surgical treatment for genital relaxation. Dr. Kegel observed that many women suffered from urinary incontinence and other pelvic floor disorders after childbirth. He created these targeted exercises to help women restore and maintain their pelvic floor strength – an oft-overlooked but critical aspect of a woman's overall reproductive health.

Over time, Kegel exercises have gained popularity as an effective and non-invasive treatment option for various pelvic floor disorders, and their remarkable benefits have been confirmed in numerous studies. Today, Kegel exercises are recommended for both men and women to enhance their overall health, with men also experiencing significant benefits in terms of prostate health and sexual function.

The Pelvic Floor: A Foundation of Strength
At the core of Kegel exercises is the pelvic floor – a group of muscles and ligaments that stretch like a hammock from the pubic bone to the coccyx (tailbone) and from one pelvic

sidewall to the other. In both genders, these muscles play a vital role in supporting the reproductive and urinary tract organs. The primary functions of the pelvic floor include:

- Supporting the pelvic organs: bladder, uterus and cervix (in women), and rectum

- Maintaining continence of urine and feces

- Facilitating sexual function

- Stabilizing the core and the spine

Pelvic Floor Disorders: Loss of Vitality and Function

As with any muscle group in the body, the pelvic floor muscles can be weakened or injured due to an array of factors. Some of the most common causes of pelvic floor dysfunction include:

- Aging

- Pregnancy and childbirth (in women)

- Obesity

- Chronic coughing or straining (e.g., during bowel movements or while lifting weights)
- Pelvic surgeries in both men and women

When the pelvic floor becomes weak, a host of problems can emerge, from urinary incontinence and pelvic organ prolapse to reduced sexual satisfaction and chronic pain. These issues can greatly impact an individual's quality of life, often leading to emotional stress and lowered self-esteem.

The Power of Kegel: Restoring Balance and Well-Being

Thankfully, Kegel exercises offer an effective solution for preventing and treating many of these pelvic floor disorders. By consistently engaging and strengthening the pelvic floor muscles through Kegel exercises, individuals can experience the following benefits:

- Improved bladder and bowel control, reducing or eliminating incontinence

- Enhanced sexual function and satisfaction

- Reduced risk of pelvic organ prolapse (in women)

- Alleviation of lower back pain and core stabilization

- Support and recovery after childbirth (in women)

- Easier and more controlled bowel movements

- Improved prostate health (in men)

1.2 Why Is Kegel Exercise Important?

The importance of physical exercise for maintaining general health and well-being is globally recognized. However, not all forms of exercise receive the attention they merit, especially those targeting "unseen" muscles. One such group of muscles that often gets overlooked and undervalued is the pelvic floor. Kegel exercises, designed to target and strengthen this crucial muscular network, hence hold prime importance for overall health and wellness.

Understanding the Role of the Pelvic Floor

The pelvic floor is a group of muscles and ligaments stretching across the base of the pelvis, acting like a supportive sling for the pelvic organs, namely the bladder, rectum, and in women, the uterus. These muscles are crucial for several core bodily functions:

- Continence Control: They play a pivotal role in maintaining urinary and faecal continence. Without adequate strength in these muscles, individuals may suffer from incontinence.

- Sexual Function: In men, a strong pelvic floor contributes to erectile function and ejaculation. In women, it aids orgasmic responses and sexual sensation.

- Core Stability: The pelvic floor muscles work in synergy with the deep muscles of the back and abdomen to provide a supportive "corset" for the spine and pelvic girdle, thus contributing to overall core stability.

The Benefits of Kegel Exercises

Given the range of critical functions these muscles perform, it becomes evident why Kegel exercises are so important. Here are some key reasons:

- Preventing and Treating Incontinence: Kegel exercises strengthen the pelvic floor muscles, thereby aiding in both prevention and treatment of urinary and faecal incontinence. This can be particularly beneficial for women who have given birth and for older individuals of both genders.

- Preparing the Body for Childbirth: For expecting mothers, regular pelvic floor exercises can help the body prepare for the stresses of labour and childbirth. They can also aid in recovery after delivery, helping to improve control over bladder and bowel function and enhancing sexual health.

- Enhancing Sexual Function: By targeting the muscle group that plays a key role in sexual function, Kegel exercises can enhance sexual health, improving sexual experience and satisfaction.

- Boosting Core Stability: Since pelvic floor muscles form a part of the inner core, Kegel exercises aid in improving core stability and strength. This can enhance overall bodily function, posture, and help prevent or manage lower back pain.

- Managing Prostate Health in Men: For men, particularly those recovering from prostate surgery, Kegel exercises can aid in regaining bladder control. They're also used in managing symptoms of an enlarged prostate (BPH) and reducing symptoms of prostate inflammation (prostatitis).

Consistency Is Key: The Ongoing Practice of Kegel Exercises

Practising Kegel exercises regularly allows individuals to maintain a strong pelvic floor, resulting in improved function and reduced risk of dysfunction. It's important to note that like any other form of exercise, the benefits of Kegel exercises come with consistency and perseverance. Regular, ongoing practice is necessary to achieve and maintain results.

Being straightforward to perform, Kegel exercises can easily be integrated into daily routines and require no specialized equipment. Despite their simplicity, their impact on quality of life can be profound, especially for individuals who may have been suffering in silence from the effects of pelvic floor dysfunction.

In essence, the importance of Kegel exercises lies in their empowering ability to give individuals back control over their bodies, improving self-esteem, personal comfort, and overall health and wellness.

Chapter two
Kegel Exercises Explained

2.1 Defining Kegel Exercises

Kegel exercises, whether discussed in hushed tones or touted as essential wellness practices, are fundamentally power practices focused on strengthening the pelvic floor muscles. These key muscles are vital for numerous functions, from holding our internal organs in place to controlling the flow of urine and faeces to contributing to sexual performance and pleasure. As such, the significance of Kegel exercises cannot be overstated.

The Origins: Naming and Purpose

Kegel exercises are named after Dr. Arnold H. Kegel, an American gynaecologist who, in the early 1940s, first introduced these exercises as a non-surgical approach to preventing 'genital relaxation,' a phrase he used to describe weakened pelvic muscles. Dr. Kegel intended these exercises mainly as a method for women to regain control over their bladder, particularly post-childbirth, when some women struggle with urinary incontinence.

The Anatomy: Pelvic Floor Muscles

The pelvic floor muscles are the group of muscles that Kegel exercises target. These muscles are like a hammock and stretch from the pubic bone in front to the tailbone (coccyx) in the back and span sideways across the base of the pelvis. They support the bladder, rectum, and in women, the uterus and vagina.

In essence, the healthy functioning of our urinary and digestive systems (and in women, the reproductive system) depends on the tonicity and strength of these crucial muscles.

The Performance: How to Do Kegel Exercises

Performing Kegel exercises primarily involves contracting and relaxing the pelvic floor muscles. Here are some general steps:

1. Identify the Correct Muscles: To do this, try stopping your urine flow mid-stream the next time you go to the bathroom. The muscles you use are your pelvic floor muscles.

2. Contract the Muscles: Tighten (contract) your pelvic floor muscles as if you're trying to hold in urine or gas. Do not bear down, squeeze your buttocks or thighs, hold your breath, or exert pressure on your abdominal muscles. The contraction should be purely focused on the pelvic floor muscles.

3. Hold and Release: Hold the contraction for about five seconds (or as many as you can muster to begin with) and then relax for five seconds. Try to

increase the hold time gradually as your muscles strengthen.

4. Repeat and Regularize: Aim for at least three sets of 10-15 repetitions a day. Consistency is key, as the benefits of Kegel exercises come with regular and extended performance.

2.2 The Science Behind Kegel

Understanding the science behind Kegel exercises is crucial in recognizing their importance and effectiveness for a range of health conditions and general well-being. These simple yet effective exercises target the pelvic floor muscles, a group of muscles that, despite their critical role in various bodily functions, often receive minimal attention.

Foundations: The Pelvic Floor Anatomy

To understand the science of Kegel exercises, it's essential to first understand the anatomy they target. The pelvic floor is a structure composed of muscles and connective tissues that extends like a hammock from the pubic bone at the front to the base of the spine at the back. It supports crucial organs such as the bladder, the bowel, and in women, the uterus.

These muscles have several vital functions:

1. Support: The primary function of the pelvic floor muscle is to hold the organs of the pelvis in place. Weakness or damage in these muscles can result in pelvic organ prolapse, where organs like the uterus or bladder descend and protrude into the vagina.

2. Continence Control: The pelvic floor muscles, in conjunction with sphincter muscles, control the excretion of urine and faeces. Their weakness can lead to incontinence (unwanted leakage).

3. Sexual Function: In men, the pelvic floor muscles are responsible for erectile function and ejaculation. In women, they contribute to sexual sensation and arousal.

4. Stability and Posture: As part of the "core" muscles, the pelvic floor muscles work in conjunction with the deep back and abdominal muscles to stabilize the body and maintain posture.

The Science of Kegel Exercises: Muscle Training

Kegel exercises are essentially a form of training for the pelvic floor muscles. Just like any other muscle in your body, the pelvic floor muscles can be strengthened and toned through targeted exercises.

The basic execution of a Kegel exercise involves repeatedly contracting and relaxing these muscles. This exercise can be performed anywhere and at any time, as it doesn't require any special equipment. The muscles you use to stop your urine flow mid-stream are essentially the pelvic floor muscles, and the act of contracting them is the basic Kegel exercise.

Physiological Impact of Kegel Exercises

Regularly performing Kegel exercises leads to an improvement in the strength and endurance of the pelvic floor muscles. Here's a detailed look at the physiological impact:

1. Muscle Hypertrophy: Just as weight lifting promotes muscle growth (hypertrophy) in the arms and legs, repeated and resisted contraction of the pelvic floor muscles can lead to increased bulk and power.

2. Improved Blood Flow: Regular exercise of any muscle group enhances blood flow to the exercised region. Increased blood supply to the pelvic area,

therefore, can help improve sexual function and speed up postpartum recovery in women.

3. Neurological Adaptation: Much like other forms of strength training, performing Kegel exercises involves both voluntarily contracting the muscles and improving mindfulness of the muscle group. This increased awareness, a form of neurological adaptation, can lead to improved control over the muscles, thereby helping to manage incontinence.

Quantifiable Improvement: The Science of Results

Numerous scientific studies back the effectiveness of Kegel exercises. Research has shown a significant improvement in urinary and faecal incontinence in both men and women following a regimen of Kegel exercises. Notably, they are also recommended for pregnant women to reduce the risk of incontinence post-childbirth and for men suffering from prostate issues.

In the realm of sexual health, both women and men have reported enhanced sexual function following regular pelvic floor muscle training. Some studies have indicated improvement in erectile dysfunction and premature ejaculation in men, along with increased arousal and orgasmic response in women.

Thus, the science behind Kegel exercises reveals them as a powerful tool for enhancing pelvic floor muscle health, setting a foundation for better urinary and faecal control, improved sexual health, and overall improved quality of life.

2.3 History of Kegel Exercises

Kegel exercises are recognized worldwide for their array of health benefits, particularly in areas often left undiscussed, such as urinary incontinence, sexual health, and pelvic floor strength. Despite their prevalence in modern health advisories with universal acceptance, the origin and history of Kegel exercises aren't as widely known.

The Birth of the Kegel Exercise

Kegel exercises are named after Dr. Arnold H. Kegel, an American gynaecologist who lived in the first half of the 20th Century. Dr. Kegel first introduced these exercises during the 1940s as a method of controlling incontinence in women after childbirth. These exercises, a new approach to 'genital relaxation', were designed to strengthen the pelvic floor muscles, thereby protecting women from the weaknesses that childbirth can introduce.

The Work of Dr. Arnold H. Kegel

Dr. Kegel's career was largely spent investigating the anatomy and physiology of the female pelvic floor, mainly focusing on managing urinary incontinence. He aimed to develop a non-surgical approach to improve the condition, an approach that would give power back to the patients, enabling them to take control of their rehabilitation.

During his studies, Dr. Kegel noticed that women who performed these exercises had a stronger pelvic floor, leading to better control over bladder function. This observation prompted him to devise an exercise regime, which now bears his name, that could be used to strengthen the pelvic floor muscles.

The Introduction of the 'Kegel Perineometer'

Dr. Arnold Kegel also invented a device called the 'Kegel Perineometer,' which was meant to measure the strength of a woman's pelvic floor muscles. By inserting the device into the vagina, one could measure the pressure within the vagina, reflecting the strength of the surrounding muscles. Dr. Kegel used this instrument to monitor the progress of his patients and validated the effectiveness of the Kegel exercises. As such, the perineometer played a key role in the development and popularization of Kegel exercises.

Expansion Beyond Women's Health

Initially, Kegel exercises were primarily recommended for women, particularly those recovering from childbirth. However, over time, the scope of these exercises expanded. By the latter half of the 20th century, it was recognized that Kegel exercises could benefit men as well, primarily those recovering from prostate surgery.

Today, these exercises are recommended for people of all genders and ages, aiding in managing conditions such as bladder and bowel incontinence, pelvic organ prolapse, and sexual dysfunction.

The Legacy and Modern Practice

Over the years, Kegel exercises have grown in popularity and are now considered a first-line approach to improving pelvic floor strength. They are widely recommended in a variety of settings, including prenatal classes, physiotherapy clinics, gynaecologist offices, and in sexual health guidance.

The enduring legacy of Dr. Kegel's exercises highlights their effectiveness and underscores the importance of pelvic floor health. The journey of Kegel exercises from a clinical prescription by a gynaecologist to a globally recognized exercise regime is testament to their utility and effectiveness.

In our modern context, where desk-bound jobs and sedentary lifestyles contribute to a general weakening of these critical muscles, Kegel exercises provide a simple, non-invasive, and practical method of maintaining and regaining pelvic floor strength. The resounding message of the history of Kegel exercises is that attention to the health of these 'hidden' muscles can greatly enhance quality of life. The tremendous work of Dr. Arnold Kegel has given us an effective tool to maintain our bodily health.

2.4 Anatomy and Physiology of Pelvic Floor Muscles

Deep within the lower body, nestled within the bony structure of the pelvis, the pelvic floor muscles surprise us with their versatile functions. These set of muscles, though inconspicuous, have a direct impact on urinary, bowel, sexual health, and more.

Anatomy of Pelvic Floor Muscles

The pelvic floor muscles, sometimes described as a 'sling' or a 'hammock', consist of layers of muscles stretching from the pubic bone in the front to the tailbone or coccyx at the back, and from one ischial tuberosity (sit bone) to the other (side-to-side).

The structures form three muscular layers stacked on top of each other:

- Superficial Layer: The muscles in this layer include bulbospongiosus, ischiocavernosus, superficial transverse perineal muscles, and the external anal sphincter.
- Middle Layer: This layer consists of the urogenital diaphragm, made up of the deep transverse perineal muscle and the sphincter urethrae.

- Deep Layer: The muscles making up this layer include the puborectalis, pubococcygeus, and iliococcygeus muscles. Together they are often referred to as the levator ani.

The pelvic floor muscles provide the base or 'floor' of the pelvic cavity and hence the name. They are tasked with housing and stabilizing several important organs, which are determined by the sex of the individual. In males, they support the bowel and bladder, whilst in females, they support the bowel, bladder, uterus, and vagina.

Physiology of Pelvic Floor Muscles

Pelvic floor muscles play a pivotal role in the following functions:

1. Support: They provide critical support to pelvic organs and also maintain intra-abdominal pressure, helping maintain the body's overall balance and posture.

2. Sphincter Mechanism: They control the opening and closing of the urethra and anus, thereby

helping in maintaining continence - control over urinary and faecal release.

3. Sexual Function: In women, contractions of the pelvic floor muscles are responsible for the pleasurable sensations of orgasm. In men, they contribute to erection and ejaculation.

4. Pregnancy and Childbirth: In women, the pelvic floor muscles help in childbirth. They provide support to the fetus and help in maintaining the optimal positioning of the baby during pregnancy. They also facilitate in the birthing process.

Conditions Associated With The Pelvic Floor Muscles

Understanding the anatomy and physiology of pelvic floor muscles provides insights into several health conditions that may arise due to their dysfunction. These conditions include but are not limited to:

- Urinary Incontinence: This can result from weak pelvic floor muscles where they cannot support the bladder properly or control the release of urine.

- Pelvic Organ Prolapse: In women, weakened pelvic floor muscles may result in the descent or dropping of the pelvic organs into or through the vagina.

- Sexual Dysfunction: Weakness or tightness of the pelvic floor muscles can contribute to erectile dysfunction in men and painful intercourse in women.

- Lower Back Pain: Since the pelvic floor muscles play a role in stabilizing the pelvis, their weakness can contribute to lower back pain or other postural issues.

The Significance of Pelvic Floor Health

A properly functioning pelvic floor is crucial for maintaining urinary and faecal continence, enjoying a fulfilling sexual life, contributing to core stability, and in women, carrying a pregnancy healthily and recovering postpartum.

As such, activities and exercises such as Kegels that aim to strengthen the pelvic floor muscles can profoundly impact one's quality of life. These exercises, which involve contracting and relaxing the pelvic floor muscles, can be incorporated into daily routines by individuals of any gender for promoting overall pelvic health.

Chapter three

Benefits of Kegel Exercises

3.1 Immediate and Long-Term Benefits

Pelvic floor exercises, most famously known as Kegel exercises, have gained significant attention over the past several decades for providing a range of health benefits. As mentioned in previous responses, the pelvic floor is a group of muscles that play a pivotal role in an individual's overall health and well-being. Engaging in pelvic floor exercises helps to maintain and optimize the function of these powerful muscles. By exploring both short-term and long-term benefits, we can better appreciate the importance of these exercises.

Immediate Benefits of Pelvic Floor Exercises

Regular practice of pelvic floor exercises provides a wide range of instant benefits, which include:

- Increased Pelvic Floor Muscle Awareness

  As you practice pelvic floor exercises, you develop a greater understanding and heightened awareness of the pelvic muscles. This familiarity with the muscle group can lead to improved muscle control, which is particularly useful for managing incontinence and other related issues.

- Improved Blood Flow

  Much like any other form of exercise, engaging the pelvic floor muscles increases blood flow to the region, nourishing the tissues and promoting muscle health.

- Enhanced Stability and Posture

  Pelvic floor exercises can provide immediate improvements to posture and stability. The pelvic floor, when tight and strong, works in harmony with the other core muscles to maintain your balance and support your spine.

- Stress Relief

  Like any form of physical activity, engaging in pelvic floor exercises can help alleviate stress and enhance relaxation, primarily due to the release of endorphins and increased blood flow.

Long-Term Benefits of Pelvic Floor Exercises

Incorporating pelvic floor exercises as a routine practice promotes numerous long-term benefits and protects the body from various health issues. The following are some of the most important long-term benefits:

- Improved Continence Control

  Regular pelvic floor exercises strengthen the muscles responsible for controlling the flow of urine and faeces. This helps in minimising accidental leaks or unwanted releases, thereby preventing or ameliorating urinary and faecal incontinence.

- Prevention and Management of Pelvic Organ Prolapse

Strengthening the pelvic floor muscles through exercise can help prevent or reduce the risk of pelvic organ prolapse. This condition occurs when the pelvic organs descend due to weakened muscles. Pelvic floor exercises can, therefore, provide much-needed support to these organs and minimize the risk of prolapse.

- Enhanced Sexual Health

Pelvic floor muscle training has been shown to improve sexual function in both men and women. In women, stronger pelvic floor muscles can lead to increased arousal, more pleasurable sensations, and more satisfying orgasms. Similarly, men can benefit from improved erectile function, better ejaculation control, and enhanced sexual performance.

- Pregnancy and Postpartum Support

For pregnant women, having strong pelvic floor muscles can be invaluable during pregnancy and the postpartum period. Strong muscles in this area can help prevent or manage incontinence during pregnancy and after childbirth, facilitate smoother labor, and aid in the recovery process post-delivery.

- Reduced Back Pain and Injury Risk

By supporting the spine and abdomen, a strong pelvic floor reduces the risk of lower back pain and injuries related to bodily instability. This is particularly significant for individuals who engage in physically demanding tasks or those with pre-existing musculoskeletal issues.

3.2 Kegel Exercises for Men and Women

Kegel exercises, designed to strengthen the pelvic floor muscles, are a simple yet effective exercise that can provide numerous health benefits. Primarily developed to aid women recovering from childbirth, the versatility and effectiveness of Kegel exercises have led to their widespread use among both men and women. Despite their universal benefits, the approach and emphasis can differ between genders due to the anatomical and physiological differences in the pelvic regions of men and women.

Kegel Exercises for Women

In women, the set of muscles composing the pelvic floor supports the uterus, bladder, small intestine, and rectum. However, factors like pregnancy, childbirth, ageing, and being overweight can weaken these muscles over time.

Kegel exercises can help address this weakness, providing the following benefits:

- Preventing Urinary Incontinence: Regular practice of Kegel exercises can prevent or alleviate urinary incontinence, which is often a problem experienced after childbirth or during menopause.

- Support During Pregnancy: During pregnancy, there's a significant increase in pressure on the pelvic muscles. Performing these exercises helps strengthen the muscles, which can make delivery easier and assist with recovery postpartum.

- Enhancing Sexual Pleasure: By increasing the strength and tone of the pelvic floor muscles, women can experience enhanced sexual pleasure and more intense orgasms.

To perform the exercises, women are instructed to tighten the muscles they would use if they were trying to stop the flow of urine. Once identified, the process includes contracting these muscles, holding for a few seconds, and then relaxing them.

Kegel Exercises for Men

While Kegel exercises are often associated with women, they are equally important and beneficial for men. The pelvic floor muscles in men provide support to the bladder and bowel and play a role in sexual function. Here are some of the benefits Kegel exercises can offer men:

- Control of Urinary and Fecal Incontinence: For men experiencing urinary or faecal incontinence, regular Kegel exercises can help improve muscle control and reduce or eliminate leaks.

- Erectile Function and Sexual Performance: By enhancing muscular control and increasing blood flow, Kegel exercises can provide benefits such as longer-lasting erections and improved sexual performance.

- Prevention and Recovery from Prostate Surgery: For men undergoing prostate surgery, Kegel exercises can aid in both preventing associated complications and facilitating faster recovery post-surgery.

3.3 Kegel Exercises and Sexual Satisfaction

Kegel Exercises and Sexual Satisfaction

When it comes to maintaining and improving sexual health and satisfaction, exercising the pelvic floor muscles by performing Kegel exercises can play a pivotal role. These powerhouse muscles are not only responsible for bodily support and continence control, but also have a significant impact on sexual function and pleasure for both men and women. In this section, we will delve into the relationship between Kegel exercises and sexual satisfaction, exploring the benefits it offers each gender and providing guidelines to enhance your overall sexual experience.

The Link Between Kegel Exercises and Sexual Satisfaction Kegel exercises, designed by Dr. Arnold Kegel in the 1940s, sought to strengthen the pubococcygeus (PC) muscles of the pelvic floor in women after childbirth. However, through the years, the importance of strong pelvic floor muscles in men has also been recognized for its significant impact on sexual performance.

In both sexes, the pelvic floor muscles help control contractions that occur during orgasms, as well as erections and ejaculation in men. Consistent Kegel exercises can greatly improve the tone, strength, and function of these muscles, resulting in heightened sexual satisfaction and performance.

Sexual Benefits of Kegel Exercises for Women

The practice of Kegel exercises can provide several sexual benefits for women, including:

- Increased Sexual Arousal: Stronger pelvic floor muscles lead to increased blood flow to the area, which in turn can heighten sexual sensitivity, arousal, and lubrication.

- Enhanced Orgasms: Consistent Kegel exercises result in stronger muscle contractions during orgasm, intensifying the pleasurable sensations experienced.

- Improved Sexual Control: A strong pelvic floor allows for better control over the vaginal muscles, enabling women to actively engage in sexual activity and even perform specific techniques that can enhance the pleasure for both partners.

- Reduced Pain: Kegel exercises can help to alleviate pain or discomfort during intercourse by improving overall pelvic floor muscle functionality and flexibility. This is particularly beneficial for women who experience conditions like vaginismus or dyspareunia.

Sexual Benefits of Kegel Exercises for Men

Kegel exercises can offer numerous sexual advantages for men, including:

- Improved Erectile Function: Practicing Kegel exercises can improve blood flow and muscle control, contributing to firmer, longer-lasting erections.

- Delayed Ejaculation: Men who perform Kegel exercises regularly often experience better control over their ejaculation, delaying climax if desired and potentially improving sexual encounters for both partners.

- Intensified Orgasms: Kegel exercises lead to stronger pelvic floor muscle contractions during orgasm, resulting in more intense sensations.

- Recovery from Prostate Surgery: For men who have undergone prostate surgery or suffer prostate-related issues, Kegel exercises can aid in the rehabilitation process, helping to restore sexual function more rapidly.

Tips for Practicing Kegel Exercises for Enhanced Sexual Satisfaction

Here are some guidelines to consider when utilising Kegel exercises to boost sexual performance and pleasure:

- Identify the Correct Muscles: The first step to effective Kegel exercises involves locating and isolating the correct muscles. For both men and women, these are the same muscles used to stop the flow of urine mid-stream.

- Establish a Routine: Consistency is key when practising Kegel exercises. Aim to perform these exercises daily, with a goal of three sets of 10-15 repetitions per set.

- Proper Technique: Focus on tightening your pelvic floor muscles while keeping the surrounding muscles in your buttocks, thighs, and abdomen relaxed. It's crucial to ensure you're not holding your breath during the process. Breathe normally and maintain a consistent rhythm.

- Track Progress: Keeping a personal log of your Kegel exercise routine and improvements in sexual function can serve as a source of motivation and help you stay committed to your pelvic floor strengthening journey.

- Patience is Essential: Remember, progress takes time. It might be several weeks or even a few months before you begin to see noticeable improvements in sexual function or pleasure. Stick with it and allow your body the time it needs to get stronger.

Chapter four

Getting Started with Kegel Exercises

4.1 How to Perform a Kegel Exercise

Kegel exercises, named after Dr. Arnold Kegel, are an essential way to strengthen the pelvic floor muscles that support our vital organs. These simple exercises can be done anywhere and offer numerous benefits such as improved bladder and bowel control, reduced risk of pelvic organ prolapse, and enhanced sexual health. Performing Kegel exercises correctly is the key to maximizing their benefits and ensuring good pelvic health. This chapter offers a comprehensive guide on performing Kegel exercises and developing a suitable routine to achieve the desired results.

Step 1: Identifying the Pelvic Floor Muscles

The first and most crucial step in performing Kegel exercises is identifying the right muscles to target. These muscles form a hammock-like structure, stretching from the pubic bone to the coccyx (the base of the spine) and from one sit bone to the other.

To locate the pelvic floor muscles, try stopping urination midstream or tightening the muscles that prevent flatulence. Make sure not to engage other muscles, such as the abdomen, buttocks, or thighs, during this process. Keep in mind that stopping urination midstream should only be done initially to locate the muscles and not as part of regular Kegel exercises, as it can lead to urinary tract issues.

Step 2: Perfecting the Technique

Now that the correct muscles have been identified, practice proper technique. Here's a step-by-step guide on how to perform a Kegel exercise:

- Contract: Contract the pelvic floor muscles as if trying to hold back urine or prevent flatulence. Be careful not to engage muscles in the abdomen, buttocks, or thighs.
- Hold: Hold the contraction for at least 3-5 seconds (or as long as possible if you're a beginner). As you become more adept, you can work up to holding the contraction for 10 seconds.
- Relax: Relax the pelvic floor muscles for an equal amount of time as the contractions (for example, relax for 5 seconds if you hold the contractions for 5 seconds). Make sure to give your muscles time to recover before the next contraction.

- Breathe: Remember to breathe normally throughout the exercise. Avoid holding your breath, as it can cause increased intrabdominal pressure and work against the desired effects.

Step 3: Establishing a Routine

Developing a consistent exercise routine is essential for reaping the full benefits of Kegel exercises. Here are some tips for setting up a successful Kegel exercise routine:

- Repetitions: Aim to perform 10-15 Kegel exercises per session. If you're a beginner, start with a lower number and gradually increase it as you build strength in your pelvic floor muscles.

- Frequency: Try to practice Kegel exercises at least three times a day to see noticeable improvements in pelvic floor strength.

- Variety: Incorporate both quick contractions (squeezing and releasing rapidly) and slow contractions (holding the squeeze for a few seconds) to target different muscle fibers.

- Consistency: As with any exercise, consistency is the key to success. Make a conscious effort to perform Kegel exercises regularly, making them a part of your daily routine.

- Tracking Progress: Monitor your progress over time. As your pelvic floor muscles become stronger, you'll be able to hold contractions for longer and perform more repetitions.

Extra Tips for Performing Kegel Exercises

1. Discretion: Kegel exercises can be performed discreetly, allowing you to practice them anywhere, anytime, such as while working at a desk or sitting in traffic.

2. Posture: Ensure good posture while doing Kegel exercises. Sit or stand upright, with shoulders

relaxed and chest open, to help facilitate proper muscle engagement.

3. Gradual Progression: As you become more adept at Kegel exercises, try increasing the duration and intensity of contractions and working up to performing more repetitions.

4. Professional Advice: Consult a healthcare professional or pelvic floor specialist if you have difficulty identifying or engaging your pelvic floor muscles or experience discomfort while performing Kegel exercises.

4.2   Understanding Your Body's Signals

Our body is an intricate and incredible machine. It continuously sends us signals that provide essential information about our physical and emotional well-being. These subtle cues can help us remain in tune with our body to prevent potential health issues, recover from injuries, manage stress, and maintain optimal functioning. Learning to understand, interpret, and respond to our body's signals is crucial for leading a healthy and balanced lifestyle. This section explores various aspects of body signals, focusing on how to recognize and react to them for better overall health.

Types of Body Signals

Our body communicates with us through various types of signals. These can generally be categorized into physical sensations, emotional responses, and changes in behaviour.

Physical Sensations

Physical sensations include pain, fatigue, hunger, thirst, and sleepiness, among others. Some common examples are:

- Pain: The body's way of signalling injury, inflammation, or an underlying health issue.
- Fatigue: Indicates the need for rest or sleep, or signals underlying medical conditions.
- Hunger: Signals an empty stomach or a dip in blood sugar levels, indicating the need for nourishment.
- Thirst: Indicates dehydration or the body's need for water to maintain its proper functioning.
- Sleepiness: A cue for the body's need to recharge, both physically and mentally.

Emotional Responses

Emotional responses encompass feelings of happiness, sadness, anger, and anxiety. They can help us recognize situations that require attention or a change in approach. For example:

- Happiness: A reward for behaviours that promote well-being, such as spending time with loved ones or engaging in fun activities.
- Sadness: Indicates a need to process emotional pain and signals a time for rest, reflection, and support from others.
- Anger: Can reveal unresolved issues, social injustice, personal boundaries being crossed, or unmet expectations.
- Anxiety: A warning that something might be amiss or a reaction to stress and uncertainty.

Changes in Behavior

Alterations in behaviour, like changes in appetite, sleep patterns, and energy levels, can signal underlying issues that may need to be addressed. Such changes could signify hormonal imbalances, chronic stress, or other health concerns.

How to Understand Your Body's Signals

Recognizing and responding to your body's signals involves cultivating self-awareness, mindfulness, and open-mindedness.

Develop Body Awareness

Body awareness entails being attentive to sensations, feelings, and physical experiences. You can develop body awareness by:

- Practising mindfulness meditation: Focus on your breath, body sensations, and thoughts during meditation to enhance self-awareness.

- Noticing physical sensations: Pay attention to sensations like pain, fatigue, hunger, and thirst, and consciously respond to these signals.

- Engaging in mindful movement: Activities such as yoga, tai chi, and dance can improve mind-body connections and help you become more aware of your body.

Keep a Journal

A journal can help track various aspects of your daily life, such as:

- Mood and emotions

- Sleep patterns

- Exercise routines

- Diet and nutrition

- Energy levels

By recording this information regularly, you can identify patterns, correlations, and potential concerns that require further attention.

Seek Professional Advice

If you're struggling to interpret your body's signals or address specific concerns, seek help from healthcare professionals or mental health specialists. They can provide guidance, insights, and support to help you gain clarity and manage your physical and emotional well-being better.

Responding to Your Body's Signals

Once you have recognized and understood your body's signals, it's essential to respond appropriately.

Self-Care

Prioritize self-care to maintain your physical and emotional health:

- Ensure adequate sleep
- Eat a balanced diet
- Stay hydrated

- Exercise regularly

- Manage stress through relaxation techniques, such as deep breathing exercises, meditation, or mindfulness practices

Set Boundaries

Establish healthy boundaries in both your personal and professional life to safeguard your physical and emotional well-being.

Seek Support

Reach out to friends, family, or support groups to share your experiences and gain insights from others in similar situations.

Make Adjustments

Make necessary adjustments to your lifestyle based on your body's signals:

- Modify your exercise routine if you notice persistent fatigue, pain, or injury.

- Adjust your diet if you experience constant hunger or changes in appetite.

- Seek medical help if you notice prolonged fatigue, persistent or severe pain, or significant changes in sleep patterns or behaviour.

4.3 Kegel Exercises for Beginners

Kegel exercises are specifically designed to strengthen the pelvic floor muscles, which support your bladder, bowels, and uterus in women and prostate in men. These simple yet highly beneficial exercises are easy to do, discreet, and require no equipment, making them a popular choice for people of all ages, especially women post-childbirth and people with urinary incontinence. As a beginner, starting a Kegel exercise routine can seem intimidating, but with patience and consistency, you can master these exercises and experience their numerous benefits.

Understanding the Pelvic Floor Muscles

Before you begin practising Kegel exercises, it's essential to understand the pelvic floor muscles. Imagine your pelvic floor muscles as a small trampoline, with the front anchored to your pubic bone and the back to your tailbone. These muscles cradle the bladder, bowels, and (in women) the uterus, controlling their functions and contributing to sexual health and core stability.

Identifying the Pelvic Floor Muscles

The first step in performing Kegel exercises is to locate your pelvic floor muscles correctly. You can identify these muscles by trying to stop your urine flow mid-stream. The muscles you engage to do this are your pelvic floor muscles. Remember, this method is only for identifying the correct muscles and not a routine exercise, as regularly stopping urine flow can lead to urinary tract issues.

Basic Kegel Exercises for Beginners

Once you've identified your pelvic floor muscles, you can start practicing Kegel exercises. Here is a simple guide for beginners:

1. Contract and Relax

- Contraction: Lie down comfortably on a flat surface with your knees bent. Tighten your pelvic floor muscles, hold the contraction for 5 seconds (or as long as you're comfortable), ensuring not to hold your breath or tighten your abdominal, thigh, or buttock muscles.

- Relaxation: Relax the muscles for 5 seconds.

- Repetition: Repeat this process 10 times. This counts as one set.

2. Quick Flicks

Aside from the longer contractions, performing 'quick flicks' can also help strengthen your pelvic floor muscles.

- Flicks: Quickly tighten and release your pelvic floor muscles, doing as many repetitions as you can manage before feeling tired.
- Breaks: Take a break for a few seconds after each bunch of 'flicks.'

3. Progression

As you gain more control and your muscles become stronger, gradually increase the contraction and relaxation intervals to 10 seconds, doing 10 repetitions for each set. Attempt to do at least three sets a day.

Tips for Performing Kegel Exercises

While the concept of Kegel exercises is simple, performing them correctly and consistently can be challenging, especially as a beginner. Here are a few tips to help you get started:

- Consistency is Key: The key to reaping the benefits of Kegel exercises is consistency. Set a regular schedule for your exercises, such as upon waking up, during lunch breaks, and before sleeping.

- Discretion: Kegel exercises can be done anywhere and in any position – sitting, standing, or lying down – as they're discreet and don't require any equipment.

- Breathe Normally: During the exercises, ensure you're breathing freely. Holding your breath can inadvertently lead to engaging your abdominal muscles, which we want to avoid.

- Don't Overdo It: If you overwork your pelvic floor muscles, you may experience fatigue and increased tension in the area. Like any other muscles, your pelvic floor needs time to recover after a workout.

Making Kegel Exercises a Routine

Creating a routine for your Kegel exercises can help ensure you perform them consistently:

In the Morning

Integrate Kegel exercises into your morning routine to start your day actively. You can do your exercises in bed before getting up or while having breakfast.

During Daily Activities

Link your Kegels to daily activities. For example, you could do a set during commercial breaks while watching TV or while waiting for your coffee to brew.

Before Bed

Performing Kegels can become a quiet, calming activity before bedtime, helping you unwind and relax.

4.4 Advanced Kegel Exercise Techniques

Kegel exercises are a well-known method for strengthening the pelvic floor muscles, providing benefits such as improved bladder control, enhanced sexual function, and a more robust core. While many people are familiar with the basic Kegel exercises for beginners, there are advanced techniques that you can incorporate into your routine to amplify the benefits and further challenge your pelvic floor muscles. This guide will outline advanced Kegel exercise techniques and provide tips for effectively integrating them into your existing routine.

Transitioning from Basic to Advanced Techniques
Before moving on to advanced Kegel exercises, make sure you've already mastered the basic techniques. This includes locating your pelvic floor muscles, performing contraction and relaxation exercises correctly, and being

able to engage these muscles without straining other muscle groups.

Advanced Kegel Exercise Techniques

Once you have a solid foundation in basic Kegel exercises, you can begin incorporating advanced techniques to enhance your pelvic floor muscles' strength and endurance further.

1. Tailor your Kegel Routine to Your Fitness Level

Now that you're more confident in your pelvic floor musculature, you can adjust the repetitions, hold durations, and frequency of your Kegels based on your current fitness level. For instance:

- Increase the contraction time to 10-15 seconds.
- Perform 15-20 repetitions per set.
- Complete 3-5 sets per day, gradually progressing as your strength and endurance improve.

2. Elevator Kegels

Elevator Kegels involve contracting and lifting your pelvic floor muscles in stages, akin to stopping at different "floors" in an elevator. This exercise helps you gain better control and awareness of your pelvic floor.

- Start by contracting your pelvic floor muscles gently, imagining you're stopping at the first floor of an elevator.
- Gradually increase the intensity of the contraction, pausing at each imaginary floor, until you reach your maximum contraction at the "top floor."
- Once you've reached the peak contraction, slowly reverse the process, releasing your pelvic floor muscles floor by floor, until you reach the "ground floor."
- Repeat this exercise 5-10 times.

3. Active Kegels

Performing Kegels during everyday activities or various exercise movements can help you build a strong pelvic floor that remains engaged even under dynamic conditions.

- Integrate Kegel exercises into activities like walking, squatting, or lunging.

- Make sure you maintain proper form and don't overly strain your buttocks, thighs, or abs while engaging in active Kegels.

- Start by holding a contraction for a few seconds during a single movement and gradually increase the hold duration as your pelvic floor becomes stronger.

4. Resistance Kegels

Adding resistance to your Kegel exercises can help increase your pelvic floor muscle strength more efficiently.

There are various pelvic floor exercisers and devices available on the market:

- Vaginal cones: Weighted cones that you insert into the vagina for women, where you engage your pelvic floor muscles to hold the cone in place.

- Pelvic floor trainers: Resistance devices that provide feedback and targeted resistance to help you perform Kegel exercises more effectively.

- Consult with a healthcare professional or pelvic floor physiotherapist before using any resistance devices to ensure their safety and appropriateness for your specific needs.

Tips for Advanced Kegel Exercises

As you progress in your Kegel journey, keep the following tips in mind:

- Maintain proper form: Stay focused on using the proper technique and avoid straining other muscle groups, such as your abs, buttocks, or thighs.

- Vary your routine: Mix up your Kegel exercise techniques to keep your muscles engaged and to prevent boredom or plateaus.

- Listen to your body: Pay attention to how your body feels during and after Kegel exercises. If you experience discomfort or pain, reassess your technique and consult with a healthcare professional or pelvic floor physiotherapist if needed.

- Celebrate progress: Acknowledge and celebrate the improvements you experience, such as better bladder control or enhanced sexual function, as you progress in your pelvic floor strengthening journey.

Persistence Pays Off

Integrating advanced Kegel exercise techniques into your routine can significantly enhance the benefits you experience from these pelvic floor-targeting exercises. Remember that progress takes time, patience, and consistency. Listen to your body and adjust your routine based on your specific needs and goals. With dedication and persistence, you'll continue to reap the rewards of a strong and healthy pelvic floor.

Chapter five

Perfecting Your Kegel Exercise Routine

5.1 Tips and Tricks for Consistency and Progress

Achieving and maintaining optimal pelvic health is within our power, thanks to practices like Kegel exercises. Named after Dr. Arnold Kegel, these exercises involve contracting and relaxing the pelvic floor muscles, providing beneficial results not limited to just improving bladder and bowel function, but extending to enhanced sexual health and bodily control. However, gaining the full benefits of Kegel exercises requires consistency and progressive effort. Here, we offer useful tips and tricks aimed at helping you enhance consistency and make significant progress in your

Kegel exercise routine, therefore, unlocking the power within.

Understanding Kegel Exercises and Their Benefits

Before delving into how to maintain consistency and progress, let's comprehend the value of Kegel exercises: Strengthen Pelvic Floor Muscles: These exercises strengthen your pelvic floor muscles, a significant factor helping with bladder control and sexual performance.

- Improved Bowel Control: Consistent practice can lead to improved bowel health and function.

- Enhanced Sexual Performance: Regular performing of Kegels can improve sexual health, heighten arousal, and enhance orgasms.

- Reduced Pelvic Pain: Kegels can alleviate discomfort associated with conditions like prolapse and endometriosis.

- Childbirth and Postnatal Recovery: For expectant mothers, regular Kegel exercises can aid childbirth and enhance postnatal recovery.

Consistency in Kegel Exercises

Understanding the need for consistency and knowing how to maintain it can make all the difference. Here's how:

Setting Realistic Goals

- Define Your Goals: Determine why you want to practice Kegel exercises and what benefits you hope to gain.

- Set Achievable Targets: Aim for a manageable number of reps and sets per day, gradually increasing as your muscles strengthen.

Establishing a Suitable Routine

- Regular Practice: Consistency is key when it comes to Kegel exercises. Set aside specific times each day for your routine.

- Flexibility: If you miss a session, don't stress. Resume wherever possible and maintain the routine afterwards.

Forming Habits

- Associate with Everyday Tasks: Link your Kegel exercises to daily tasks like brushing your teeth, having a meal, or while doing household chores.
- Use Reminders: Set reminders on your phone or write it on your calendar until it becomes a habit.

Progressing in Kegel Exercises

Seeing progress in your Kegel exercise practice is crucial to motivate you to continue. Here's how you can fuel your growth:

Monitoring Your Improvement

- Track Your Progress: Note down the number of repetitions, sets, and hold-duration for each exercise session and monitor the improvement over time.

- Reflect on Changes: Consistently observe and reflect on how your body is reacting to the exercises, noticing improvements in bladder control or bowel function.

Continuous Learning

- Stay Informed: Stay updated on new techniques or variations that can make your Kegel practice more effective.

- Participate in Workshops: Join workshops or seminars that focus on pelvic health to learn from experts and gain more insights.

Overcoming Obstacles in Kegel Exercises

Staying consistent and progressing in your Kegel practice may pose challenges. Here's how you can overcome them:

Ensuring Proper Technique

- Check with a Professional: If unsure whether you're doing Kegels correctly, don't hesitate to consult with a healthcare professional.
- Use Biofeedback Devices: If appropriate, consider biofeedback devices that can help ensure you're contracting the right muscles.

Dealing with Lack of Routine

- Reschedule: If you tend to forget to do your exercises, reschedule them to a time when you're less likely to be distracted.
- Commit to Consistency: Decide now that your pelvic health is a priority and commit to your exercise schedule.

Seeing Slow or No Progress

- Be Patient: Results from Kegel exercises can take weeks or even months to notice. Don't be disheartened and remain consistent.

- Seek Professional Guidance: If you're not seeing any progress after several weeks, consider seeking the guidance of a pelvic floor therapist.

5.2 Addressing Common Mistakes and Misconceptions

Kegel exercises, originally developed by Dr. Arnold Kegel, are simple clench-and-release exercises designed to strengthen the pelvic floor muscles and provide various health benefits. These exercises have garnered huge popularity due to their myriad benefits, including improved bladder and bowel control, enhanced sexual performance, and reduced pelvic pain. However, like any other practice, Kegel exercises are subject to several common mistakes and misconceptions that may impede their effectiveness. This section aims to clarify these misunderstandings and correct the common errors, allowing you to unlock your potential to the fullest through these exercises.

Common Misconceptions About Kegel Exercises

Here, take a look at some of the most common misconceptions surrounding Kegel exercises and the truth behind them.

"Only Women Need to Do Kegel Exercises"

Contrary to popular belief, Kegel exercises are beneficial for both men and women. Men can also suffer from weak pelvic floor muscles, which can lead to problems like urinary incontinence and sexual dysfunction. Kegel exercises can effectively combat these issues.

"Doing Kegels Can Result in Over-Tightening of Pelvic Muscles"

While it's important to exercise caution, Kegel exercises done correctly and in moderation will not cause your pelvic muscles to become too tight. Instead, they will build strength and flexibility in these muscles and lead to improved control.

"Kegel Exercises are Unnecessary if You're Young and Healthy"

Pelvic floor muscles can weaken due to a variety of reasons, not just age or poor health. Pregnancy, childbirth, surgery, heavy lifting, and excessive straining can all lead to pelvic floor dysfunction, regardless of age or health status. Proactive exercises like Kegels can help maintain optimal pelvic floor health.

Common Mistakes While Doing Kegel Exercises

Despite their apparent simplicity, Kegel exercises involve several nuances and require proper technique. Here are some common mistakes that practitioners need to avoid for effective results.

Incorrect Identification and Engagement of Muscles

One of the biggest mistakes while performing Kegel exercises is incorrect identification and engagement of the pelvic muscles. Engaging the wrong muscles, such as the abdomen, buttocks, or thigh muscles instead of the pelvic floor muscles, can render the exercises ineffective and even put undue strain on these areas.

Holding the Breath

Many people unconsciously hold their breath while performing Kegel exercises. However, it's crucial to breathe normally during the exercises, as holding the breath can put pressure on the pelvic muscles, defeating the purpose of the exercise.

Over-exercising

Just like any other muscle group, over-exercising the pelvic floor muscles can lead to muscle fatigue and strain. It's important to start with a manageable routine and slowly increase the frequency and intensity of the exercise over time.

Addressing These Mistakes and Misconceptions

Understanding and rectifying these errors and misconceptions is crucial to ensure the optimal effectiveness of Kegel exercises.

Seeking Professional Guidance

One of the best ways to avoid mistakes and correct misunderstandings is to seek professional guidance. A healthcare professional or pelvic floor therapist can provide accurate information and practical guidance to ensure proper form and technique.

Using Biofeedback Devices

Biofeedback devices, widely used in physical therapy, can be effectively used to identify the correct muscles for Kegel exercises. These devices provide visual or auditory feedback to help you understand whether you're engaging the right muscles.

Regular Monitoring and Adjustment

Once you've started performing Kegel exercises, it's necessary to regularly monitor your progress and adjust your routine accordingly. Reflecting on changes in your control and strength can help you understand if you're performing the exercises correctly and making progress.

5.3 Kegel Exercise Routine for Busy People

We live in a fast-paced world, wherein busyness has gradually evolved into a state of normalcy. Regardless of their field, individuals often find themselves juggling various responsibilities, leading to bustling schedules that leave little room for self-care and health practices such as Kegel exercises. Despite the hustle and bustle, it's essential to remember that our health must never take a back seat. This guide is specially designed to help busy individuals incorporate a convenient and comprehensive Kegel exercise routine into their daily lives.

Understanding Kegel Exercises

Named after Dr. Arnold Kegel, these exercises focus on strengthening the pelvic floor muscles, leading to benefits like improved bladder and bowel control, enhanced sexual health, and stronger muscular control. The exercises simply involve the contraction and relaxation of these muscles in a controlled manner.

Schedule-Friendly Kegel Exercise Routine

For those juggling busy schedules, finding a workout routine that fits seamlessly into their daily lifestyle is vital. The following Kegel exercise routine is crafted keeping in mind this very need, offering flexibility and ease of practice.

Morning Kegels

Fit your first set of exercises in the morning as part of your routine.

- Ideally, practice them after your morning bathroom routine when your bladder is empty to avoid discomfort.

- Aim for 10 quick contractions and releases, followed by 10 slow ones where the hold lasts for about 5 seconds.

Mid-day Kegels

The beauty of Kegels is that they can be done discreetly, meaning you can fit a set in during a work break.

- Carry out the same routine as in the morning: 10 quick Kegel exercises and 10 slow ones.
- It might be helpful to set a reminder on your phone initially until it becomes a habit.

Evening Kegels

As you wind down your day, find some time before bed for the last set of exercises.

- Like the previous sets, aim for 10 quick contractions and releases, and then 10 slow ones.
- Try to relax and breathe deeply during this session, using it as a time of mindful relaxation as well.

Tips to Efficiently Incorporate Kegels into Your Daily Routine

Here are some additional tips to integrate Kegel exercises into your busy schedule effectively:

- Associate with Everyday Tasks: Link Kegels with routine tasks. This could be while brushing your teeth, during a TV commercial, or while waiting for the microwave to beep.

- Use Reminders: Until your Kegel exercises become a habit, use reminders on your phone or sticky notes around your household/workplace.

- Keep it Simple: Do not worry about the exact number of sets you perform each day while starting out. The aim initially is to get used to the exercises and remember to include them in your daily routine.

- Do Them Anywhere: Since Kegel exercises do not require special equipment and are not noticeable, take advantage of time spent waiting, such as in traffic, queues, or on hold during a phone call.

Monitoring Progress

To benefit from this schedule, consistency is key. Regularly practising Kegels will strengthen your pelvic floor muscles over time, giving you the desired results. Keep track of how many Kegels you can do initially and how long you can hold them. Over time, aim to increase both the number of repetitions and the hold duration, while ensuring your technique is appropriate.

5.4 Using Kegel Exercise Equipment and Apps

Kegel exercises entail a simple rhythmic contracting and releasing of the pelvic floor muscles to bolster the muscles' strength, control, and flexibility. While these exercises can be performed without any tools or technological assistance, employing equipment and apps can provide additional benefits such as expert guidance, real-time feedback, and increased motivation. This section delves into the various types of Kegel exercise equipment and apps available that can make your exercise regimen more productive and engaging.

Kegel Exercise Equipment

There are several devices on the market specifically designed to aid Kegel exercises by providing targeted resistance, enhanced engagement, and real-time feedback. Highlighted below are some of the popular types of equipment.

Kegel Weights

These weighted devices, also known as vaginal weights, vaginal Cones, or Ben Wa balls, are inserted into the vagina and serve as a resistance tool for pelvic floor muscles during Kegel exercises. The goal is to contract the muscles and keep the weight in place. Available in different sizes and weights, they can be tailored according to user preference and experience.

Biofeedback Devices

Biofeedback devices monitor and measure muscle activity, relaying visual or auditory feedback to help users understand and control pelvic floor contractions. These devices can be inserted or used externally and, when connected to an app, can provide reporting data or progress tracking.

Kegel Exercisers

These devices are specially designed to apply direct pressure to pelvic floor muscles, allowing for more precise and active engagement. Usually shaped like a probe or clamp, Kegel exercisers come in various designs and offer different degrees of tension. Some models come with built-in biofeedback mechanisms or app connectivity to enhance the exercise experience.

Kegel Exercise Apps

In addition to equipment, several mobile apps can help guide, track, and motivate your Kegel exercise routine. Here are some popular features found in Kegel exercise apps:

Guided Exercise Sessions

Many Kegel apps offer structured exercise sessions that guide users through variations of contractions, holds, and relaxation patterns. These routines can be personalized to fit individual needs and progress.

Reminders and Scheduling

One of the challenges faced by those performing Kegel exercises is remembering to practice consistently. Kegel exercise apps often have scheduling options that send reminders or alerts to ensure regular exercise.

Progress Tracking

Kegel apps help to monitor user progress over time by maintaining logs of exercise sessions, sets, repetitions, and hold durations. Users can analyze their progress, identify potential issues, and tailor their workouts accordingly.

Gamification

To keep users engaged, many Kegel apps use gamification techniques, including achievements, challenges, and rewards. Such methods have been found to enhance motivation and adherence to exercise regimens.

Connectivity with Compatible Devices

Some Kegel exercise apps work in tandem with compatible devices, such as biofeedback devices or Kegel exercisers. The app collects data from these devices during exercise sessions and uses it to provide real-time feedback, allowing users to tweak their contraction strength and technique.

How to Choose the Right Equipment and App

When selecting Kegel exercise equipment or apps, bear in mind the following factors:

- Ease of Use: Consider equipment and apps that are user-friendly and easy to clean, ensuring that it is simple to incorporate into daily routines.
- Compatibility: Ensure the chosen equipment is compatible with the app to maximize its utility.

- Personalization: Opt for tools that allow for customization, enabling users to adapt exercises to their unique needs and progress.

- Privacy: When using mobile apps, be cautious about privacy, checking if permissions and data usage policies align with personal comfort levels.

- Medical Advice: Consult a healthcare professional for guidance on choosing the most appropriate Kegel exercise equipment and app for individual circumstances.

Chapter six

Special Considerations for Kegel Exercises

6.1 Kegel Exercises During Pregnancy and Postpartum

Kegel exercises, also known as pelvic floor muscle training, play a critical role in preparing the body for the changes it will go through during pregnancy and childbirth. Postpartum, these exercises also help in the recovery process. This comprehensive guide will delve into the significance of Kegel exercises during pregnancy and postpartum, outlining how and when to do them, as well as their benefits.

Understanding Kegel Exercises and the Pelvic Floor

Kegel exercises target the muscles in your pelvic floor, a "hammock-like" structure that supports the uterus, bladder, small intestine, and rectum. Maintaining the strength and flexibility of these muscles is paramount for pregnant women to ease childbirth, and after delivery, to promote healing.

Benefits of Kegel Exercises During Pregnancy

During pregnancy, the body experiences significant changes, including weight gain, shifts in the centre of gravity, and hormonal fluctuations. These changes put considerable pressure on the pelvic floor muscles. Kegel exercises are beneficial because:

- Improved Childbirth Experience: Strong pelvic floor muscles can ease labour and delivery. Women who regularly do Kegel exercises may find it easier to push during the birth process.

- Reduced Risk of Incontinence: The added weight of pregnancy can strain pelvic muscles, causing bladder leaks. Kegel exercises strengthen these muscles, improving bladder control.

- Relief from Hemorrhoids: Regular Kegels can help reduce the risk of developing haemorrhoids, common during pregnancy.

Benefits of Kegel Exercises During Postpartum Recovery

Kegel exercises also offer numerous benefits postpartum, including:

- Improved Pelvic Floor Recovery: Childbirth can weaken and stretch the pelvic floor muscles, leading to challenges like incontinence and lowered sexual satisfaction. Regular Kegel exercises can aid in the recovery and toning of these muscles.

- Supports Healing After a Tear or Episiotomy: Practicing Kegel exercises can improve blood circulation to the perineal region, promoting healing after an episiotomy or perineal tear.

- Enhanced Sexual Satisfaction: The tightening and relaxing of pelvic muscles during Kegel exercises can improve sensation during sexual activities.

When to Start and How to Perform Kegel Exercises

You can start practising Kegel exercises at any stage of your life, but they are particularly beneficial when started in early pregnancy and continued throughout the postpartum period. Here's how you do them:

- Locate Your Pelvic Muscles: These are the muscles that you use when trying to stop the flow of urine midstream or hold in gas.

- Contract and Hold: Tighten these muscles, hold for 5-10 seconds, then relax. Repeat this sequence in sets of 10.

- Stay Focused: Try not to involve your abdominal, buttock, or inner thigh muscles. The focus should be solely on the pelvic muscles.

- Consistency is Key: Practice Kegel exercises at least three times a day.

It may take time to see results, so don't be disheartened if improvement isn't immediate. Your consistency and persistence will pay off.

Safety Measures and Precautions

While Kegel exercises are generally safe during pregnancy and postpartum, it's always wise to consult a healthcare provider before starting any new exercise regimen. Some precautions include:

- Don't Overdo It: Overworking your pelvic muscles by performing Kegels too frequently or holding your contractions for too long can lead to straining and discomfort.

- Avoid Holding Your Breath: Remember to breathe normally during the exercises. Holding your breath can result in an increase in abdominal pressure.

- Postnatal Care: After delivery, consult your healthcare provider before starting or continuing your Kegel exercise routine, particularly if you've had a cesarean delivery or pelvic complications.

6.2 Kegel Exercises for Age-Related Changes

As people age, their muscles and connective tissues often become weaker. This is true for the pelvic floor muscles as well. The weakening of the pelvic floor muscles can lead to various health issues, such as urinary incontinence, bowel dysfunction, and pelvic organ prolapse. Kegel exercises, also known as pelvic floor muscle training, can play a crucial role in addressing age-related changes.

This guide will discuss in detail the importance of Kegel exercises for managing the age-related changes in the pelvic floor muscles, the benefits of these exercises, and how to perform them correctly and safely.

Understanding Age-Related Pelvic Floor Changes

Age-related changes in the pelvic floor muscles can be attributed to factors like:

- Natural loss of muscle mass and strength
- Decrease in hormone levels (e.g., estrogen in women)
- Obesity, which adds pressure on the pelvic floor
- Previous pregnancies and giving birth vaginally
- Chronic constipation or straining during bowel movements
- History of pelvic surgeries

- Chronic coughing due to smoking or respiratory conditions

These factors result in the weakening of pelvic floor muscles, leading to common issues such as urinary incontinence, faecal incontinence, and pelvic organ prolapse.

Benefits of Kegel Exercises for Age-Related Changes

Kegel exercises help strengthen the pelvic floor muscles, providing numerous benefits for people experiencing age-related pelvic floor changes:

1. Improved Urinary Incontinence: Strengthening the pelvic floor muscles can lead to better bladder control, reducing the chances of stress, urge, or mixed incontinence.

2. Better Bowel Control: Kegel exercises can help improve rectal muscle tone, minimising faecal incontinence and other bowel dysfunctions.

3. Reduced Pelvic Organ Prolapse: Regular Kegel exercises can support prolapsed pelvic organs and delay the progression of pelvic organ prolapse.

4. Enhanced Sexual Function: Strong pelvic floor muscles can result in increased blood flow and sensitivity in the genital area, leading to improved sexual sensation and function.

5. Support for Prostate Health: For men, Kegel exercises can help alleviate some symptoms related to prostate enlargement, such as frequent or urgent urination.

6. Strengthened Core: Keeping the pelvic floor muscles strong can contribute to overall core strength, promoting better balance and stability.

How to Perform Kegel Exercises Correctly

1. Locate the Pelvic Floor Muscles: To identify these muscles, try to stop the flow of urine midstream or squeeze your anal muscles as if trying to prevent passing gas. These are the muscles you need to work on.

2. Empty Your Bladder: Make sure to perform Kegel exercises with an empty bladder.

3. Begin with Slow Contraction: Tighten your pelvic floor muscles, hold the contraction for about 5 seconds, then relax for another 5 seconds. As you get more comfortable, gradually increase the contraction time to 10 seconds and the relaxation time to 10 seconds.

4. Complete Multiple Repetitions: Aim to perform 10 to 15 repetitions per session, and work up to 3 sessions daily.

5. Consistency: Practicing Kegel exercises regularly is the key to experiencing their benefits. Be patient, as it may take several weeks or months of consistent practice to notice significant improvements.

6. Breathing: Breathe evenly and avoid holding your breath while performing the exercises.

Safety Tips and Precautions

1. Consult Your Healthcare Provider: It's essential to speak with your healthcare provider before starting Kegel exercises, especially if you have existing pelvic health concerns.

2. Don't Strain: Avoid straining or holding your breath during the exercises, as this can put additional pressure on your abdominal and pelvic floor muscles.

3. Technique Matters: Performing Kegel exercises
   with incorrect technique won't help improve your
   pelvic floor muscles and may even cause harm.
   Ask your healthcare provider or a pelvic floor
   specialist to ensure proper technique.

4. Avoid Overtraining: Like any other muscle group,
   overworking your pelvic floor muscles may lead to
   fatigue, soreness, or even injury. Stick to the
   recommended frequency and intensity of the
   exercises to prevent overtraining.

6.3 Kegel Exercises for Medical Conditions

Kegel exercises, or pelvic floor muscle training, are often advocated for their myriad benefits related to pregnancy and postpartum recovery. However, what many people might not be aware of is their remarkable effectiveness in managing certain medical conditions. By strengthening the pelvic floor muscles, Kegel exercises can alleviate symptoms associated with several common disorders, ranging from urinary incontinence to erectile dysfunction. This guide will delineate the healing power of Kegel exercises in combatting certain medical conditions, illustrating their fundamental role in fostering healthier and more comfortable living.

Understanding Kegel Exercises

Introduced by Dr. Arnold Kegel, Kegel exercises are subtle movements designed to strengthen the pelvic floor muscles. These are the muscles that support the bladder, uterus, rectum, and small intestine. By tightening and relaxing these muscles, you can improve their strength and endurance.

Kegel Exercises for Various Medical Conditions

Kegel exercises emerge as an effective non-surgical treatment for various medical conditions, with a broader application than just improving pregnancy outcomes. Let's look at some of these conditions where Kegel exercises can provide significant symptomatic relief:

1. Urinary Incontinence

Urinary incontinence refers to the loss of bladder control, causing involuntary leaks of urine. It's widespread in both males and females, especially the elderly. Kegel exercises can fortify the muscles that control urinary flow, improving bladder control, and reducing or even eliminating incontinence.

2. Faecal Incontinence

Similar to urinary incontinence, fecal incontinence is a condition that results in accidental bowel leakage. The causes vary, but often it's due to weakened rectal muscles.

Kegel exercises can strengthen these muscles, leading to improved bowel control.

3. Overactive Bladder

An overactive bladder can cause an urgent desire to urinate, even when the bladder isn't full. This abrupt urge can sometimes lead to involuntary loss of urine. By bolstering the pelvic floor muscles, Kegel exercises can help manage these sudden urges and serve as an effective treatment for the condition.

4. Pelvic Organ Prolapse

In this condition, one or more of the pelvic organs (including the bladder, uterus, or rectum) collapse into or protrude out of the vagina. This is often due to weak pelvic floor muscles. Regular Kegel exercises can help to hold these organs in place and alleviate symptoms associated with pelvic organ prolapse.

5. Erectile Dysfunction and Premature Ejaculation

In men, Kegel exercises can aid in achieving and maintaining penile erection – the challenge lying at the heart of erectile dysfunction. These pelvic exercises can also help control ejaculation, providing an effective strategy for coping with premature ejaculation.

How to Perform Kegel Exercises

Performing Kegel exercises is quite easy:

1. Identify your pelvic floor muscles: The easiest way to do this is by trying to stop your urine flow midstream. The muscles used to do this are your pelvic floor muscles.

2. Contract and relax: Contract these muscles for 5-10 seconds, then completely relax them for about the same duration. This contracts-relaxes cycle constitutes one repetition.

3. Repeat: Aim for at least three sets of 10 repetitions per day.

Remember, Kegels should not cause pain. If you experience any discomfort while doing these exercises, you're likely using incorrect technique or straining too hard. Consult with a healthcare provider to ensure that you're performing them correctly.

Precautions and Safety Measures

Before you rush to start your regimen of Kegel exercises, it's important to be aware of several measures to ensure safety:

1. Consult with your healthcare provider: Before starting Kegel exercises, specifically for managing

medical conditions, it's advisable to consult with your healthcare provider.

2. Learn correct technique: Doing Kegel exercises incorrectly can make your symptoms worse. It's very beneficial to learn the correct technique, ideally under professional supervision.

3. Don't overdo it: Avoid the urge to practice Kegel exercises more frequently or intensely than recommended, as overworking your pelvic muscles can actually lead to muscle fatigue and worsening of symptoms.

4. Relaxation is key: After each contraction, it's important to fully relax your pelvic muscles. If you skip this relaxation phase, the exercises might not be as effective.

Chapter seven

Conclusion

7.1 Final Thoughts

This journey into the world of Kegel exercises — their mechanisms, applicability, and benefits — illuminates their extraordinary potential and transformative power. These simple yet potent exercises offer a safe, cost-effective, and non-surgical avenue for addressing numerous common health complaints that can drastically impact quality of life.

The ubiquity of conditions like urinary incontinence, faecal incontinence, overactive bladder, and pelvic organ prolapse underscores the urgency of obtaining widespread awareness about Kegel exercises. Beyond mere treatment, Kegels offer a powerful preventive strategy —

strengthening the pelvic muscles and maintaining pelvic fitness can fend off several of these disorders.

Even more transformative is Kegel's potential power in matters of sexual health. The effectiveness these exercises have shown in managing erectile dysfunction and premature ejaculation positions them as a promising, non-pharmacological approach to enhance sexual wellbeing in men. This can have profound implications not only for individual self-esteem and relationship satisfaction, but also for overall mental health.

Importantly, the practice of Kegel exercises is uncomplicated and accessible. They require no specialized equipment or dedicated space, nor do they demand extensive time — making them easy to incorporate into daily routines. However, this apparent simplicity should not eclipse the importance of correct technique and careful execution. Consulting with a healthcare provider or a pelvic floor specialist can be invaluable in instilling the right exercise habits early on.

The versatility of Kegel exercises and their scope of application across genders and ages underscore their potential to enhance and safeguard health, from pre-pregnancy to golden years. However, Kegels are not a panacea. While they possess vast health potential, they may not serve as the exclusive solution for all pelvic health issues. It's essential to remember that individual health needs vary, and in some cases, additional treatments may be necessary.

Despite their relative obscurity outside of the domain of pregnancy and postpartum care, the conversation around Kegel exercises is gaining momentum in broader healthcare spheres. This is both remarkable and necessary. By unlocking the power within our bodies — the power of Kegels — we can all strive towards better health, improved comfort, and enhanced living.